UNLOCK THE POWER
OF LYCOPENE

SO-AGH-400

by David Yeung, Ph.D.,
Venket Rao, Ph.D., and
Idamarie Laquatra, Ph.D., R.D.

Introduction by Maureen Storey,
Center for Food, Nutrition and Agriculture Policy, University of Maryland

Published by arpr, inc.

Important Notice

The material contained in this book is for informational purposes only. It is not meant to function as a prescription or to substitute for the advice of a medical professional. Persons who have cancer, heart disease or other medical conditions should be guided by the direction and advice of their medical professionals. Good nutrition and sound dietary habits are not substitutes for treatment by a medical professional. Specifically, the consumption of lycopene and tomato products must not be substituted for the direction and advice of your medical professional. The authors and publisher disclaim and shall not be liable or responsible for any use, misuse or applications of this book to treat, diagnose or medicate a medical problem, disease or other condition.

Unlock the Power of Lycopene – Revised 2nd Edition
Redefining Your Diet with Lycopene and Tomatoes

For information or inquiries address: arpr, inc., 2213 Centre Avenue, Suite 2216, Pittsburgh, PA 15219 USA

ISBN: 0-9773839-0-3

For information or inquiries, visit: www.lycopene.org

Printed in the United States of America
arpr, inc. paperback edition/September 2005

Library of Congress Control Number: 2005934613

Yeung, David, 1939-
    Unlocking the power of lycopene: redefining your diet for optimum health/by David Yeung and Venket Rao.
        p. cm.
    Includes bibliographical references and index.
    ISBN 0-977389-0-3 (pbk.)
    1. Tomatoes — Health aspects. 2. Lycopene — Health aspects. I. Rao, Venket, 1936- II. Title

Table of Contents

Introduction

It is my great pleasure to introduce you to the updated, second edition of *Unlock the Power of Lycopene, REDefining Your Diet with Lycopene and Tomatoes.*
As the director of the Center for Food, Nutrition and Agriculture Policy at the University of Maryland, what and how we eat is of great personal and professional interest to me, and has been the main focus of my career for the past two decades. With childhood and adult obesity, cancer rates and other health ailments associated with unhealthy lifestyles, it is critical that we reverse these trends.

As such, the research being conducted on the antioxidant lycopene—found in fresh and processed tomato products—will help us understand its potential health benefits.

This updated version of *Unlock the Power of Lycopene* contains all the original background information about tomatoes, their storied history, many interesting facts about tomatoes and the numerous nutrients they provide. It also includes new information about ongoing research, the updated food pyramid, the potential health benefits of lycopene, and many new and tasty recipes for incorporating tomatoes into your diet in new and interesting ways.

Tomatoes are an integral part of a Mediterranean-style diet; one rich in fruits, vegetables, grains and olive oil, and low in saturated fat, which is central to reducing the risk of heart disease, cancer and other health problems. *Unlock the Power of Lycopene* provides a solid basis of information about this important antioxidant in our daily lives.

I hope this book provides not only the basis for learning why it's so important to incorporate tomato lycopene into your daily diet, but also the encouragement and the ways to do so. I wish you many years of healthful eating.

Dr. Maureen Storey

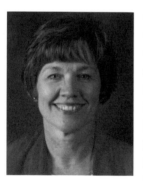 *Dr. Maureen Storey is Director and Research Professor of the Center for Food, Nutrition and Agriculture Policy (CFNAP)—a newly created independent, affiliated center in the Division of Research at the University of Maryland, College Park. She is also Deputy Director of the University of Maryland/U.S. Food and Drug Administration's Joint Institute for Food Safety and Applied Nutrition (JIFSAN). Dr. Storey is a member of the American Society for Nutritional Sciences, the Institute for Food Technologists and the American Dietetic Association.*

CHAPTER ONE

Fruits, Vegetables and Health

How Eating Right May Help Prevent Disease

Good nutrition and regular physical activity are the keys to good health. But what exactly does "good nutrition" mean? In recent years, researchers have expanded their focus from specific nutrients to foods that contain these nutrients. And, finally, to eating patterns that incorporate food combinations that may be able to prevent or even fight serious diseases.

That's right! A dinner of spaghetti with marinara sauce and a tossed salad seasoned with olive oil, vinegar and herbs topped off with sliced fresh fruit for dessert might be a step forward in keeping your heart and blood vessels healthy. Adding a glass of tomato juice to your snack of nuts might be part of a healthy lifestyle that can help you ward off cancer.

There is growing evidence that diet, combined with other healthy lifestyle habits, plays a major role in preventing disease. For example, the Mediterranean diet is rich in fruits, vegetables, grains, and olive oil and low in saturated fat. Research shows that such a diet may help cut the risk of heart disease and cancer. The Dietary Approaches to Stop Hypertension (DASH) diet includes liberal amounts of fruits and vegetables, whole grains and low-fat dairy products, and is low in saturated and total fat. This diet is effective for preventing and treating high blood pressure.

The Mediterranean Diet[1]

Summary of dietary pattern
High intakes of fruits and vegetables (especially green leafy vegetables, tomatoes, onions, garlic), legumes, fish, cereals and nuts; moderate in fat (olive oil); low meat consumption; moderate wine consumption.

Benefits
Reduced risk of heart disease; reduced risk of cancer

Protective Nutrients
Phytochemicals, omega-3 fatty acids, vitamins and minerals

The DASH Eating Pattern[2]

Summary of dietary pattern
High intakes of fruits and vegetables; inclusion of low-fat dairy products, whole grains, poultry, fish and nuts. Reduced in fats, red meats, sweets and sugar-containing beverages.

Benefits
Lowered blood pressure

Protective Nutrients
Phytochemicals, vitamins, minerals, fiber

You will notice that the dietary patterns mentioned above contain liberal amounts of fruits and vegetables. Scientific research suggests that generous amounts of fruits and vegetables, as part of a healthy diet, help protect our bodies from many chronic diseases including stroke, heart disease, type 2 diabetes, cancers of the oral cavity, pharynx, larynx, lung, esophagus, stomach and colon-rectum[3]. In fact, most countries are now placing a stronger emphasis on fruits and vegetables. In the United States, the 2005 Dietary Guidelines list fruits and vegetables as "foods to encourage," and they are emphasized in the MyPyramid graphic that consumers can use.

Fruits and vegetables are nutrition powerhouses. They are rich sources of vitamins, minerals, fiber and natural substances known as "phytochemicals."

Phytochemicals perform a number of functions in plants, including protecting some plants from disease. There are thousands of phytochemicals, some of which have been used for hundreds of years as medicines, such as quinine for malaria and digitalis for heart conditions.

A sample of fruits and vegetables, and some of their phytochemicals and actions are listed below.

Plant	Phytochemical	Actions
Broccoli, cauliflower, cabbage	Glucosinolates: sulforaphane	Cancer preventive
Carrots, sweet potato, spinach, apricot	Carotenoids: beta-carotene	Antioxidant
Garlic, onions	Allyl compounds: allyl sulfides	Cancer preventive; lowers risk factors for heart disease
Oranges	Flavonoids: hesperetin	Possible anti-inflammatory; may lower risk for heart disease
Red grapes, berries	Phenolic compounds: ellagic acid	Cancer preventive
Tomatoes, pink grapefruit	Carotenoids: lycopene	Antioxidant, anti-inflammatory

Scientists have been especially interested in the antioxidant action of phytochemicals. Antioxidant activities may be critical in fighting many diseases, including cancer, heart disease, age-related macular degeneration, diabetes and osteoporosis. A closer look at antioxidant activity will help to explain how fruits and vegetables might be able to help fight disease.

Antioxidant Activity

Some scientists think that phytochemicals that have antioxidant activity may protect your health by fighting substances in your body called free radicals. Free radicals are unstable molecules produced during normal body metabolism and as a result of environmental factors. For example, free radicals are produced when your body burns (oxidizes) food. Like a car's engine burning gasoline and producing exhaust and pollution, this process produces a kind of internal pollution: free radicals. Indeed, pollution, smoking and other environmental factors can create more free radicals in our bodies.

Another way to think about oxidation is to understand that it is the same process that makes iron rust and fruit turn brown. It doesn't take much to see that free radicals do the same kind of damage to the cells in your body. Moreover, when a free radical attacks another molecule, it turns that molecule into another free radical. This sets off a chain reaction that creates more and more free radicals which, in turn, damage more cells. Many scientists think this cell damage may trigger a host of diseases, including cancer and heart disease.

Fortunately, phytochemicals with antioxidant activities protect us from oxidative damage. They sometimes act like bodyguards protecting cells, or they can "disarm" or neutralize free radicals before they can do damage.

Nutritionists agree that the best way to get phytochemicals is through the diet rather than by supplements[3].

Current dietary guidelines encourage an eating pattern that includes generous amounts of fruits and vegetables—nine servings daily on a 2000-calorie diet. Most people do not yet achieve the recommended intakes, but the good news is that fruit and vegetable consumption is on the rise. In the fruit category, we eat more servings of apples than any other fruit. In the vegetable category, fresh and processed tomatoes rank second only to potatoes as the most popular vegetable[4,5], and tomato consumption is expected to grow in the next decade[6].

The increasing popularity of tomatoes is thought to be because of our greater tendency to eat away from home, enjoying ethnic foods that include tomato sauces and pastes used in their preparation. Also, the public is increasingly aware of the health benefits of including processed tomato products in the diet.

In Chapters 2 and 3, we'll examine the history and characteristics of the tomato. In Chapters 4 and 5, we'll tell you more about the specific health benefits of tomatoes and processed tomato products. To help you meet the government recommendations for a healthy eating pattern that incorporates more fruits and vegetables (including tomatoes!), whole grains and low-fat dairy products into your diet, turn to Chapter 6. There you'll find daily menus with tested recipes to start you on your way to better health.

CHAPTER TWO

Tomato Tradition

*The Story of the Tomato,
from the Aztecs to Today*

Today the tomato is one of our favorite sources of
nutrition — but it faced a tough fight to be accepted
on menus in the United States, Canada, Great Britain,
much of northern Europe and Asia.

The tomato originated in the Andes Mountains in
South America, and was first domesticated in Mexico
by the Aztec people. The word "tomato" seems to be
derived from the Aztec word "tomatl." After the
Spanish conquered Mexico in the early 1500s, they
introduced it to southern Europe, where it quickly
became popular. The Italians may have called it
"pomodoro" — golden apple — perhaps because the
first tomatoes often were yellow. But others say that
the Italian name originally was "poma amoris,"
meaning "apple of love." The French also called it
the apple of love, "pomme d'amour." This name
may have been prompted by the heart shape of many
tomatoes of that era and gave rise to the legend that
the tomato was an aphrodisiac.

The tomato received a much chillier reception in colder climates, however. In parts of the United States, Canada and Great Britain, it often was called the "wolf peach." This rather unappealing name reflects the poor reputation of the tomato in those countries and throughout much of northern Europe. Many people even thought tomatoes were poisonous. This belief may have sprung from the fact that the tomato is related to poisonous plants such as belladonna and nightshade, and indeed vines and leaves of the tomato plant can be poisonous. Whatever the reason, for many years it was grown only as a decorative plant in much of North America and northern Europe.

Another reason, perhaps, for the reluctance of people in northern countries to eat tomatoes was that most diets in those regions were bland, both in taste and color. In the era before refrigeration and mass transportation, fresh fruits and vegetables were available only for short portions of the year. People used to a diet of starches and meat were slow to realize the culinary potential of the tomato's vibrant red color and resonant flavor. Nevertheless, it slowly made inroads. Thomas Jefferson grew them at his farm at Monticello as early as 1781 as a decorative plant. In the early 1800s, it began to gain some cautious acceptance in the United States.

A story illustrates the process. In Salem, N.J., about 1822, amateur horticulturist Robert Gibbon Johnson vowed to eat tomatoes on the steps of the courthouse. His own physician warned him he would "foam and froth at the mouth ... double over with appendicitis ... if [the] 'wolf peach' is too ripe and warmed by the sun ... exposing himself to brain fever." A crowd gathered to watch this horrific spectacle. Johnson went ahead and ate tomatoes from his garden. To the surprise of the townsfolk, he displayed obvious relish for the juicy red vegetables and suffered no evident side-effects. From Salem the word spread: tomatoes were not only safe, they were delicious — or so the story goes.

In any event, by the middle of the 19th century the tomato had become widely accepted in the United States and the rest of the world. One factor was the growing popularity of tomato ketchup. Ketchup has been around for centuries, though its precise origins are in dispute. It may have been created in Asia: some experts have speculated the word "ketchup" was originally a Malay word, "kitjap." At first, ketchup meant any of a wide array of sauces, including some made from walnuts, beans or anchovies. With the growing popularity of the tomato, tomato ketchup became a favorite way to add the taste and color of tomatoes to meals year-round.

Farmers and horticulturists rapidly developed the red, round tomato we see most often in our supermarkets today. In 1949, the first hybrid tomatoes appeared, aiding tomato production. For instance, in the 1960s the development of hardy breeds of tomatoes, along with the refinement of tomato-harvesting machines, aided the cultivation of processing tomatoes. The tomato crop is, after the potato crop, the most important commercial vegetable product in the United States, both in terms of how many tomatoes are grown and how many tomatoes and tomato products are consumed. It also is, according to some experts, the biggest contributor of nutrients to the American diet.

The situation is similar in other countries. Tomatoes now are grown virtually throughout the world and have revolutionized diets across the globe. The tomato has made its biggest mark in Italian, Spanish and Mexican cooking, but cooks everywhere have found it to be versatile and tasty. You could easily have a different tomato-based recipe every day of the year, with plenty left over. The tomato has found a role in an almost unlimited number of casseroles, stews and other main dishes; from shrimp jambalaya to tomato chow mein to tomato cake, not to mention a multitude of sauces and dressings.

But what lies behind its popularity? Let's find out.

CHAPTER THREE

Team Tomato

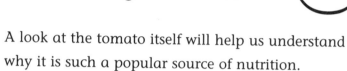

Understanding the Tomato

A look at the tomato itself will help us understand why it is such a popular source of nutrition.

Tomatoes answer to the scientific name of Lycopersicon esculentum, which roughly translates as "edible wolf peach," recalling the days it was eyed with suspicion. The tomato indeed is related to the poisonous night-shade plants, and also is part of the larger Solanaceae family, which includes potatoes, eggplant, and cayenne and tabasco peppers.

Tomatoes and tomato sauces are packed with nutri-ents, with little fat and no cholesterol. For example, 100 grams of tomato sauce has 30 calories, 1.3 grams of protein, 7 grams of carbohydrates and a little more than a gram of fiber.

Varieties

Let's look at the many different kinds of tomatoes and tomato plants.

Size. Tomatoes generally range in size from three-quarters of an inch in diameter and a quarter of an ounce in weight to six inches in diameter and two pounds, but some are much bigger. The biggest tomato on record was a seven-pound behemoth grown in Oklahoma.

Color. Tomatoes range in hue from white to red to purple, including green, yellow and orange. The lighter colors generally have a milder flavor. One note: only red tomatoes have lycopene, because lycopene is the red pigment that gives them their color.

Determinate and indeterminate plants.

"Determinate" tomato plants are rather compact bushes that grow to a certain size and then stop, with their tomatoes reaching maturity at roughly the same time. "Indeterminate" tomato plants, or vines, keep growing until the frost (or extreme heat in warmer climates) kills them.

Store tomatoes and processing tomatoes.

Store (fresh market) tomatoes are picked when they are green, because they need to ripen during the trip to market to have the best flavor. They also are picked by hand because they must be picked at just the right stage in the ripening process, and then must arrive on the shelves in perfect condition.

To give consumers the best prices and quality for sauces and ketchup, processing tomatoes must be harvested in the most efficient manner possible, and this means that the tomatoes themselves need to be different. First of all, they must be picked together at the peak of ripeness, then processed within a few hours of ripening. This means that they are grown on determinate plants that have been specially bred so that the tomatoes ripen at about the same time. Efficiency requires machine harvesting and rapid transportation, so growers have developed hardy tomatoes that can withstand being picked by machines and not be crushed when transported at the bottom of 25,000-pound truckloads, yet still have all the taste and nutrition you expect in tomato products.

Shape. The five main shapes are, in order of size, cherry, plum, pear, standard and beefsteak.

Maturity date. This is the number of days from the date of planting to the time when they can be expected to be ripe.

Flavor. Studies have shown that a substance called furenol, which develops during the ripening process, is the main source of the tomato's flavor. That is why tomatoes need to ripen to present the best taste. Also, there isn't much difference in the acidity of most kinds of tomatoes. Tomatoes that taste "less acidic" really just have more natural sugar.

The popular varieties of garden tomatoes alone number in the hundreds. To give you an idea of the tomato's many colors, sizes and flavors, here are the names of just a few of the popular tomato varieties:

Celebrity Champion	Better Boy	Bucks County
Dona	Delicious	French Rose
Early Girl	Fourth of July	Red Star
Fantastic	Tumbler	Mortgage Lifter
Golden Nugget	Medina	Lemon Boy
Jubilee	Heatwave II	Good 'n Early
Mr. Stripey	Celebrity	Garden Peach
Siberia	Red Satin	Small Fry
Sun Gold	Sweet Tangerine	Big Beef
Sweet Million	Saladette Ensalada	Best Boy
Top Sirloin	Green Grape	

Fruit or Vegetable?

There's one more way of describing tomatoes that occasionally sparks disputes: are they fruits or vegetables?

If you're like most people, you think of tomatoes as vegetables. After all, in a salad they are eaten with lettuce, green pepper, onions and other vegetables; we cook tomatoes along with other vegetables in sauces or casseroles. But if you talked to a botanist, he or she might insist that the tomato is a fruit. What's the answer? In a way, the answer is "both of the above."

In botanical terms, the tomato itself is a fruit, because a fruit is considered to be any sweet pulp containing a seed or seeds. A horticulturist, however, would say the tomato plant is a vegetable plant. That is because most "fruits" are grown on trees: think of apple, peach or cherry trees. But the tomato plant is a vine or a bush, like most of the plants you'll see in a typical vegetable garden.

In the United States, the argument has been settled by the highest court in the land. In 1893, the U.S. Supreme Court ruled on a lawsuit on that very question because, at the time, vegetables were subject to a tariff and fruits were not. "Botanically speaking," the Court ruled, "tomatoes are the fruit of a vine, just as are cucumbers, squashes, beans and peas. But in the common language of the people, whether sellers or consumers of provisions, all these are vegetables which are grown in kitchen gardens, and which, whether eaten cooked or raw, are, like potatoes, carrots, parsnips, turnips, beets, cauliflower, cabbage, celery, and lettuce, usually served at dinner in, with, or after the soup, fish, or meats which constitute the principal part of the repast, and not, like fruits generally, as dessert."

Today many people follow the Court's reasoning and call the tomato a vegetable.

Popularity

Although tomato plants generally require warm weather and lots of sunlight, they are adaptable and vigorous. This is shown by the fact that, of the nearly 30 million Americans who have gardens, perhaps as many as 95 percent of them grow tomatoes, making it the most popular home-garden vegetable in the United States. The tomato has been just as enthusiastically received in other nations, though in colder climates it usually is grown in greenhouses.

Thanks to the tomato's own adaptability, varieties, many uses, and modern development, it has become very popular. Americans consume an average of almost 90 pounds of tomatoes every year for every man, woman and child in the nation, with about 18 pounds of that as fresh tomatoes, and the rest as processed tomato products. To meet this demand, American farmers in 2004 grew more than 1.8 million tons of fresh-market tomatoes and more than 12 million tons of processing tomatoes.

Let's turn now to another source of the tomato's popularity in our health-conscious age: its many nutrients.

CHAPTER FOUR

Unlock the Power

The Tomato's Many Health Benefits

Regardless of whether the tomato is called a fruit or vegetable, it is an important component in the North American diet. Government data show the average person in the United States consumes approximately 18 pounds of fresh tomatoes, and more than 70 pounds of processed tomatoes per year, and these values are expected to increase[1]. This puts fresh tomatoes in the top five fresh vegetables most commonly consumed, and processed tomatoes at the top of the list of all processed vegetables consumed[1].

Both fresh and processed tomatoes are treasures of nutrients, with processed tomatoes having higher levels of nutrients simply because the vegetable is concentrated. Because tomatoes and tomato products are so popular, they are important contributors to vitamin and mineral intake. In fact, they are one of the top five food sources contributing to intakes of vitamin C, vitamin A, vitamin E, potassium and fiber[2].

Vitamin C

Many of us do not realize that tomatoes contribute the second highest amount of vitamin C to our diets. Orange and grapefruit juices provide the most. Vitamin C has long been known to prevent scurvy, a scourge among our ancestors when fruits and vegetables were not always available. Scurvy is a condition that is characterized by bleeding gums and soreness in the joints.

Vitamin C also is a powerful antioxidant. In nature, it helps retain the color and freshness of fruits and vegetables. In the human body, it may protect us against heart disease, certain types of cancer, cataracts, asthma and obstructive pulmonary disease. It is believed to reduce the duration and severity of the common cold in some individuals. Vitamin C also has the ability to enhance the absorption of iron from plant foods. This means that we absorb more iron in our breakfast cereal if we include a glass of tomato juice or orange juice with breakfast.

Vitamin A

Tomatoes are an important source of vitamin A in our diets. This is because tomatoes contain a high level of beta-carotene, which is converted to vitamin A in our bodies. A lack of vitamin A can lead to night blindness, which is the inability of our eyes to adapt from bright light to darkness. Extreme deprivation of vitamin A can lead to total blindness. Vitamin A also is very important for the maintenance of the skin and tissue lining, including that of the eye. Vitamin A is involved in immune function and, therefore, for the prevention of infections. Also, beta-carotene-rich diets have been associated with a lower risk of cardiovascular disease and cancer[3].

Vitamin E

Vitamin E's primary function in the body is its antioxidant activity. It targets and disrupts reactions of free radicals. It especially protects cell membranes. A deficiency of vitamin E is rare in North America. While most dietary vitamin E is found in oils and foods that contain fat, tomatoes—because of the large amount consumed—are substantial contributors to vitamin E intake.

Potassium

Potassium is an essential nutrient that is important for normal health maintenance and growth. Tomatoes rank fifth in the foods that provide potassium in our diets. In the body, potassium, as an electrolyte, is necessary for controlling the body's acid-base balance, movement of nutrients across the cell membranes, nerve conduction and muscle contraction. A deficiency of potassium can result in cramps, muscle weakness, mental confusion, apathy, anorexia and coma.

A diet rich in potassium can also lower blood pressure. A potassium-rich diet blunts the effects of salt on blood pressure, may reduce the risk of developing kidney stones, and possibly decrease bone loss with age[4].

Fiber

Tomatoes are a top contributor of dietary fiber. There are many different types of dietary fiber, and they have different beneficial effects on our bodies. Some of the actions of dietary fibers include:

- Delaying stomach emptying of foods we consume, resulting in a feeling of fullness that may help with weight management;
- Improving insulin sensitivity;
- Reducing blood cholesterol;
- Preventing constipation;
- Possibly protecting against colon cancer.

We do not get enough fiber in our diets. Current recommendations are that men should strive to include 38 grams of fiber in their diets daily, and women should aim for 25 grams. Most individuals only consume about half the recommended amount. The easiest way to include the different fibers in our diets is to consume fruits, vegetables and whole grains each day. By incorporating 2 cups of fruit and 2-1/2 cups of vegetables daily, and choosing whole grain breads and cereals to make up half of our grain servings, we can achieve dietary fiber goals and enjoy its protective effects.

Beyond Vitamins and Minerals: Phytochemicals in Tomatoes

Tomatoes are excellent sources of a good number of phytochemicals, including those classified as carotenoids and polyphenols. These phytochemicals possibly together are thought to reduce the risk of many chronic diseases.

Tomato Phytochemicals

Carotenoids
- Beta-carotene
- Alpha-carotene
- Lycopene
- Lutein + Zeaxanthin
- Phytoene
- Phytofluene

Polyphenols
- Quercetin
- Kaempferol
- Naringenin

Other Compounds
- Oligosaccharides

Lycopene

In tomatoes and tomato products, lycopene is the carotenoid in highest concentration. Lycopene is a natural red pigment that gives the tomato its typical red color. Redder tomatoes have higher levels of lycopene. Lycopene is also found in apricots and a small number of red fruits such as watermelons, pink guava, and pink grapefruit. More than 85% of lycopene in our diets comes from 10 foods[5]. These include watermelon, fresh tomatoes, and eight processed or cooked tomato products: spaghetti/pasta sauce, ketchup, salsa, tomato soup, canned tomatoes, tomato sauce, tomato paste, and vegetable juice cocktail.

Product	Lycopene mg/100g[a]	Serving Size[b]	Lycopene mg/serving
Tomato Juice (no salt added)	9.3	240 mL (1 cup)	22.9
Tomato Ketchup	17.0	15 mL (1 tbsp)	2.9
Spaghetti Sauce	16.0	125 g (1/2 cup)	20.0
Tomato Paste	29.3	30 g (2 tbsp)	8.8
Tomato Soup (condensed)	10.9	245 g (1 cup prepared)	13.1
Tomato Sauce	15.9	60 g (1/4 cup)	9.6
Chili Sauce	13.0*	15 mL (1 tbsp)	2.2
Seafood Cocktail Sauce	12.2*	60 g (1/4 cup)	7.3
Watermelon	4.9	280 g (~1/16 of a watermelon)	13.6
Pink Grapefruit	1.5	154 g (1/2 medium)	2.3
Raw Tomato	3.0	148 g (1 medium)	4.5

[a] USDA-NCC Carotenoid Database for U.S. Foods – 1998
[b] FDA Reference Amounts; Guidelines for Voluntary Nutrition Labeling of Raw Fruit, Vegetables and Fish
* H.J. Heinz analytical results

One of the few carotenoids that cannot be converted to vitamin A, lycopene is one of the most powerful antioxidants among the carotenoids. The basis of its power may be its chemical structure. Lycopene has a large number of "double bonds." These are chemical bonds in which two pairs of electrons are shared by two atoms in a molecule. Free radicals lack an electron, and they cause damage by grabbing electrons away from other molecules. Because it has many double bonds, lycopene is better able to donate an electron to free radicals, taming them and, in the process, protecting the body.

The very potent antioxidant activity of lycopene is thought to be its major role; however, evidence is accumulating that lycopene may act in other ways that help to protect us from disease. For example, lycopene interferes with the growth and proliferation of cancer cells in the prostate, breast, lung and endometrium. It may also help to decrease blood levels of cholesterol, reduce the development of disease by reducing inflammation, and improve immune function[6].

Lycopene, to be beneficial in the prevention of chronic diseases, must first be absorbed and then maintain its health properties in the body. Several factors influence the absorption and hence the bioavailability of lycopene. Lycopene is absorbed more efficiently from heat-processed tomato products than it is from fresh tomatoes. For example, lycopene from tomato paste was shown to be better absorbed than lycopene from fresh tomatoes[7]. In fresh tomatoes, lycopene is tightly bound into the tomato's cell structure.

When tomatoes are processed, the heating changes the molecular structure and releases the lycopene from that structure, making it more available. The presence of fats also facilitates the absorption of lycopene. Lycopene dissolves in fat, hence the importance of a small amount of dietary fat in the digestive process. This means that the presence of oil in spaghetti sauce increases the absorption of lycopene.

In addition to lycopene, tomatoes contain a variety of other carotenoids. As mentioned previously, beta-carotene is converted to vitamin A in the body. In addition, beta-carotene along with the other carotenoids in tomatoes exhibit distinct antioxidant properties[8].

Polyphenols

Tomatoes are also sources of polyphenols[8]. The polyphenols and various carotenoids found in tomatoes work in combination with lycopene to exert the beneficial health effects associated with consuming tomatoes[8], such as reducing the risk of heart disease, certain types of cancer, age-related macular degeneration and diabetes. Promising work is also showing a benefit of lycopene on osteoporosis prevention. The specific health benefits of tomatoes will be described in the following chapter.

Other Beneficial Components in Tomatoes

Tomatoes contain oligosaccharides, carbohydrates that are not broken down by the intestinal enzymes. However, they serve as nourishment for the "good" bacteria in the colon that help us digest food.

Preliminary research on the yellow fluid surrounding the seeds shows that it might be able, in some unknown way, to prevent blood clots and cardiovascular disease. Furthermore, the carbohydrate-binding protein in tomatoes has the highest agglutination activity of any fruit. Agglutination is the process of binding certain bacteria or foreign cells together, which is one way the body fights bacteria. It may be beneficial against inflammatory intestinal diseases and boost immunity.

Summing Up

There are many beneficial compounds in tomatoes. In addition to vitamins, minerals and fiber, tomatoes are a rich source of phytochemicals and other components scientists are just beginning to understand. Many of these nutrients and phytochemicals have antioxidant properties that seem to work in combination with lycopene to offer health benefits.

CHAPTER FIVE

Lessons in Lycopene

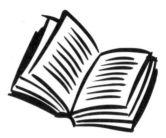

A Scientific Look at This Powerful Antioxidant in Tomatoes

The main supporting evidence for the role of lycopene in tomatoes in disease prevention comes from four kinds of scientific studies:

- Tissue culture studies that investigate how cells develop
- Laboratory studies of animals
- Epidemiological studies
- Human clinical investigations

These studies are continuing to provide a great deal of evidence for the protective effects of lycopene in tomatoes. The graph on page 30 illustrates the areas of the body that may benefit from a diet that includes lycopene in tomato products.

Following absorption of lycopene from foods, it is distributed throughout the body to various organs. Some organs, such as the prostate, liver, adrenal gland and testes, have been shown to contain much higher levels of lycopene, suggesting the presence of specialized transport mechanisms in these organs.

Every "Body" May Benefit from Lycopene

Emerging evidence shows that lycopene from processed tomatoes may reduce the risk of certain diseases within the human body.

Lycopene may benefit:

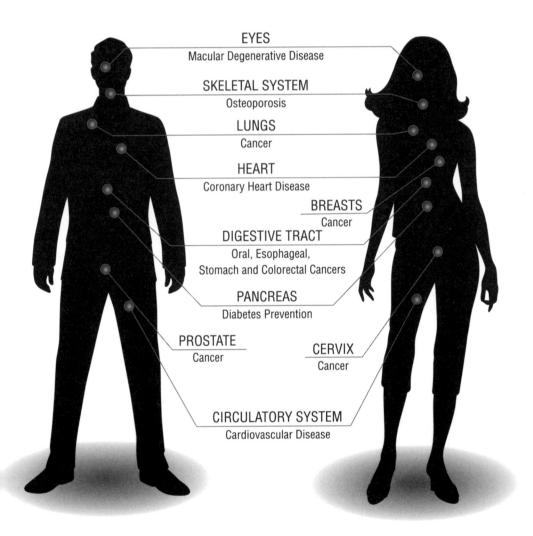

EYES
Macular Degenerative Disease

SKELETAL SYSTEM
Osteoporosis

LUNGS
Cancer

HEART
Coronary Heart Disease

BREASTS
Cancer

DIGESTIVE TRACT
Oral, Esophageal,
Stomach and Colorectal Cancers

PANCREAS
Diabetes Prevention

PROSTATE
Cancer

CERVIX
Cancer

CIRCULATORY SYSTEM
Cardiovascular Disease

Cancer

Cancer is a multistage disease in which a normal cell undergoes genetic alteration because of DNA damage. This stage is referred to as the "initiation" stage. The initiated cells then proliferate under certain conditions. The state in which cells proliferate is followed by a "progression" stage. Eventually, malignant primary tumors are formed that undergo metastasis and spread throughout the body.

Lycopene in tomato products can play an important role in fighting this process. As a potent antioxidant, it can prevent oxidative damage of the DNA and prevent the progression of cancer at its early stage. It can also battle cancer by preventing cell proliferation typical of cancer, as well as by restricting the growth of tumor cells.

Research on tomato products or lycopene and cancer is most compelling for cancers of the prostate gland, lung and stomach. Data are suggestive for pancreatic, colorectal, esophageal, oral, breast and cervical cancers. More studies are needed before making conclusive statements about other cancer sites[1].

Prostate Cancer

Prostate cancer is one of the most common cancers among men in North America. In an epidemiological study more than 20 years ago, consumption of tomato products was associated with a reduced risk of prostate cancer[2]. Men who consumed tomato products five times weekly had a significantly lower risk of prostate cancer than those who consumed less than one serving per week.

A large, comprehensive study of tomato consumption and prostate cancer risk showed that a reduced risk of prostate cancer of 35% was observed for men who consumed 10 or more servings of tomato products per week.

The protective effect was more pronounced with advanced or aggressive stages of prostate cancer[3]. Additional data from this study group more recently demonstrated that men who averaged two or more servings of tomato sauce per week had a significantly reduced risk of prostate cancer compared to men who had less than one serving per week[4].

A meta-analysis of observational studies on the role of tomato intake and lycopene in the prevention of prostate cancer further supports a protective role. It indicated that tomato intake was modestly and inversely associated with prostate cancer risk. The preventive effect was slightly stronger for cooked vs. raw tomato intake[5].

The authors of this study felt that the evidence was not strong enough to recommend lycopene supplements; in fact, the major researchers in this field recommend a diet rich in fruits and vegetables, including tomato products rather than lycopene supplements[1,6].

Animal studies have helped to define the mechanisms of action, and future studies will provide information about dose and form of tomatoes that might provide optimum cancer risk reduction[7].

Lung Cancer

The lungs are particularly at risk for oxidative stress, because they are regularly exposed to pollutants in the air. Several epidemiological studies reported a lower risk of lung cancer with greater exposure to lycopene or tomato products. Animal studies have had mixed results[8].

Stomach Cancer

Like the lung studies, epidemiological studies evaluating tomato products and lycopene related to stomach cancer show a trend toward lower risk with greater tomato product and lycopene intake[8]. Animal and clinical studies are critically needed in this area.

Other Cancers

Although limited in number, studies of the oral cavity support a reduction in risk associated with tomato consumption[1]. Research on esophageal cancers is also limited. However, a study in Iran showed a significant reduction in risk for men who consumed tomatoes frequently[9]. A study in the United States yielded a reduction, although it was not statistically significant[10].

Pancreatic cancer is a leading cause of cancer deaths, with a low survival rate. A population-based case control study completed in Canada found that lycopene intake, from a diet rich in tomatoes and tomato-based products, reduced the risk of pancreatic cancer among men by 31%[11]. This positive finding will hopefully lead to more research explaining the protective role of dietary components such as lycopene in pancreatic cancer prevention[1].

The results of epidemiological and animal studies on colorectal cancer risk and tomato products are promising[8]. Several studies support an inverse relationship between tomato consumption and colon cancer risk in men and women[6].

Cell studies and animal studies show a beneficial effect of lycopene for reducing breast cancer risk. But the few human dietary studies completed in this area have not shown an association between tomato intake and breast cancer[1]. Because breast cancer is the second leading cause of cancer-related deaths among women in North America[12,13] (lung cancer is first), more research is urgently needed.

Higher serum levels of lycopene have been associated with a lower risk of cervical cancer[8]. Few dietary studies on tomato consumption and cervical cancer are available, but they do demonstrate a positive trend between tomato consumers and reduced cervical cancer risk[1].

Cardiovascular Disease

Cardiovascular disease includes all diseases that affect the heart and blood vessel system. Heart disease is the leading cause of death in men and women in North America[14,15]. There are many theories about the cause of heart disease, but the strongest evidence exists for mechanisms involved in excess oxidative stress[16]. Free radicals cause oxidation of low-density lipoproteins (LDL), which function as the carriers of cholesterol in the bloodstream. This damage to LDL now is recognized as an important early step in the development of atherosclerosis, a hardening and narrowing of the arteries caused by the buildup of fatty plaque inside the artery walls. Dietary antioxidants, such as lycopene, may slow the progression of atherosclerosis because they can inhibit oxidative damage. In addition, lycopene may inhibit cholesterol production and enhance the breakdown of LDL[17].

Several studies now have been completed that examined blood and tissue levels of lycopene, as well as consumption of tomato products and the risk of cardiovascular disease. In a study in which subjects were recruited from

10 European countries, the relationship between antioxidant levels in fat tissue and heart attacks was examined. After adjusting for several dietary variables, only the level of lycopene was shown to protect against cardiovascular disease[18]. The authors concluded that lycopene or some other substance in a common food source was protective. In a small clinical trial, males consuming 60 mg of lycopene daily for six months showed a 14% reduction in plasma cholesterol[19].

It is possible that it is the tomato itself—not only the lycopene content—that counts. This theory is supported by a number of studies. In a study among people with type 2 diabetes, consumption of tomato juice increased plasma lycopene levels and resistance of LDL to oxidation[20].

In the Physicians' Health Study, no overall association between increasing concentrations of plasma lycopene and risk of cardiovascular disease in men was observed[21].

In the Women's Health Study, a large ongoing clinical trial, women consuming at least seven servings of tomato products weekly had a 30% reduced risk of cardiovascular disease, compared with women who had fewer than 1.5 servings per week[22]. Interestingly, in this study—although there was an association between tomato intake and cardiovascular disease—there was no overall association between dietary lycopene intake and cardiovascular disease. These findings seem to support that other tomato components work together with lycopene to offer a cardiovascular benefit.

Clearly, much more work needs to be done before conclusive statements can be made about the benefits of lycopene and tomato products in the prevention of cardiovascular disease. Well-controlled clinical intervention studies in populations at high risk for cardiovascular disease will help to clarify the role of dietary components in the prevention of this serious disease.

Other Diseases

Scientists across the world are now investigating how lycopene might help prevent other diseases and ailments. There is evidence that lycopene might help prevent age-related macular degeneration (ARMD), a disease that can lead to blindness. For example, a study at the University of Wisconsin showed that people with very low levels of lycopene in their bloodstream were more likely to get ARMD than people with higher levels[23].

It is also recognized that chronic diseases such as diabetes and osteoporosis are related to oxidative damage. Investigations on the effectiveness of lycopene in reducing the risk of these diseases are continuing. In a major study in the United States, scientists discovered that the amounts of lycopene and beta-carotene were, on average, highest in people with normal glucose tolerance, slightly lower in people with impaired glucose tolerance, and lowest in people with newly diagnosed diabetes[24].

Osteoporosis is a major public health threat in North America. Osteoporosis is the thinning and weakening of bones, making them more susceptible to fracture. Animal studies investigating the effect of lycopene on the activity of bone cells indicate that lycopene may inhibit the activity of bone cells responsible for breakdown and resorption of bone[25]. These preliminary results suggest a possible role for lycopene in the prevention of osteoporosis.

Research is ongoing, but there already is a great deal of evidence that lycopene has many health benefits. Good nutrition, including eating fruits and vegetables, is not a substitute for medical advice and treatment.

The basic message is simply this: something as delicious as tomato products may also be good for you. At this point, you may well agree that it would be a good idea to add a splash of bright red tomato products to your diet. But how much do you need?

Tomatoes and Lycopene in Your Daily Diet

Research in the area of tomato product consumption and lycopene has led scientists to the practice of using a lycopene dose ranging from 25–35 milligrams daily in the form of tomato products and lycopene capsules in their studies. A recently completed small study evaluated the effect of ingesting low levels of lycopene on its absorption and antioxidant properties. Lycopene at the levels of 5, 10 and 20 milligrams (about 2 to 7 tablespoons) was ingested by healthy people in the form of ketchup for two weeks. A significant increase in serum lycopene levels and a reduction in lipid oxidation were observed at all levels of lycopene intake[26]. It is possible, then, that the recommended level of lycopene consumed through tomato products can be revised to 5 to 7 milligrams to help maintain levels to deal with normal oxidative stress.

Recommendations for daily lycopene intake levels in populations at high risk for cancer, cardiovascular disease and other chronic diseases cannot be established because dosing studies have not been completed. Future studies must be undertaken in these populations to pinpoint beneficial intake levels.

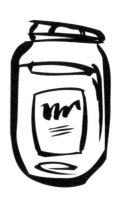

The Bottom Line

There is compelling evidence to suggest a protective role for lycopene against cardiovascular disease and a number of cancers, including prostate cancer. Evidence is also mounting in favor of lycopene in the prevention of other chronic diseases such as diabetes, age-related macular degeneration, and osteoporosis. The easiest and safest way to include lycopene in our diets is by including tomatoes and tomato products. In the next chapter, we explain current dietary recommendations for good health. We'll also provide daily menus that capture these recommendations, and provide sources of lycopene and other phytonutrients.

CHAPTER SIX

Now You're Cooking

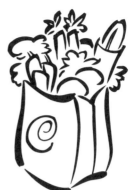

Dietary Patterns That Promote Good Health

We do not eat single nutrients; we eat foods made up of numerous nutrients. More and more, scientists are discovering that many nutrients in a single food work as a team. In addition, different foods work together to enhance health benefits. For example, we have discussed the phytochemical components in addition to lycopene in tomatoes, and how these seem to work together with lycopene to achieve health benefits.

We also know that, for example, lycopene is better-absorbed from processed tomato products and if a small amount of fat is included in the meal. Now, research supports that certain dietary patterns may be more beneficial than others.

Although much serious scientific work remains to be done in this vital and evolving area, experts agree that a poor diet and sedentary lifestyle are linked to overweight and obesity, heart disease, diabetes, high blood pressure, osteoporosis, and some types of cancer. Major efforts are

under way to help individuals improve their diets
and lifestyles.

New Dietary Recommendations

Dietary guidance from the United States Government
provides science-based advice to promote health and
reduce the risk of chronic diseases. As our understanding
of nutrients and dietary patterns improves, dietary recommendations become more detailed and complex. The
Dietary Guidelines for Americans is a perfect example.

The Guidelines began with seven guidelines in 1980,
and expanded to 10 guidelines in 2000. The 2005
Guidelines are composed of nine major areas of focus,
as well as key messages under each area:

1. Adequate nutrients within calorie needs

- Consume a variety of nutrient-dense foods and
  beverages, while choosing foods that limit the
  intake of saturated and trans fats, cholesterol,
  added sugars, salt and alcohol.
- Meet recommended intakes within energy needs
  by adopting a balanced eating pattern.

2. Weight Management

- To maintain body weight in a healthy range,
  balance calories from foods and beverages with
  calories expended.

- To prevent gradual weight gain over time, make small decreases in food and beverage calories, and increase physical activity.

3. Physical Activity

- Engage in regular physical activity and reduce sedentary activities to promote health, psychological well-being, and a healthy body weight.
- Achieve physical fitness by including cardiovascular conditioning, stretching exercises for flexibility, and resistance exercises or calisthenics for muscle strength and endurance.

4. Food Groups to Encourage

- Consume a sufficient amount of fruits and vegetables, while staying within energy needs.
- Choose a variety of fruits and vegetables each day.
- Consume 3 or more whole grain products per day.
- Consume 3 cups per day of fat-free or low-fat milk, or equivalent milk products.

5. Fats

- Consume fewer than 10% of calories from saturated fatty acids and fewer than 300 mg/day of cholesterol, and keep trans fatty acid consumption as low as possible.
- Keep total fat intake between 20–35% of calories, with most fats coming from sources of polyunsaturated and monounsaturated fatty acids, such as fish, nuts and vegetable oils.

- When selecting and preparing meat, poultry, dry beans, and milk or milk products, make choices that are lean, low-fat or fat-free.
- Limit intake of fats and oils high in saturated and/or trans fatty acids, and choose products low in such fats and oils.

6. Carbohydrates

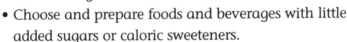

- Choose fiber-rich fruits, vegetables and whole grains often.
- Choose and prepare foods and beverages with little added sugars or caloric sweeteners.
- Reduce the incidence of dental caries by practicing good oral hygiene, and consuming sugar- and starch-containing foods and beverages less frequently.

7. Sodium and Potassium

- Consume less than 2300 mg of sodium per day (approximately 1 tsp of salt).
- Choose and prepare foods with little salt. At the same time, consume potassium-rich foods, such as fruits and vegetables.

8. Alcoholic Beverages

- Those who choose to drink alcoholic beverages should do so sensibly and in moderation (up to 1 drink daily for women and 2 drinks daily for men).
- Alcoholic beverages should not be consumed by some individuals, including those who cannot restrict their alcohol intake, women of childbearing

age who may become pregnant, pregnant and
lactating women, children and adolescents, individuals taking medications that can interact with
alcohol, and those with specific medical conditions.
- Alcoholic beverages should be avoided by individuals
engaging in activities that require attention, skill, or
coordination, such as driving or operating machinery.

9. Food Safety

To avoid microbial foodborne illness:
- Clean hands, food contact surfaces, and fruits and
vegetables. Meat and poultry should not be rinsed.
- Separate raw, cooked and ready-to-eat foods while
shopping, preparing or storing foods.
- Cook foods to a safe temperature to kill
microorganisms.
- Chill (refrigerate) perishable food promptly and
defrost foods properly.
- Avoid raw (unpasteurized) milk or any products
made from unpasteurized milk, raw, or partially
cooked eggs or foods containing raw eggs, raw, or
undercooked meat and poultry, unpasteurized
juices, and raw sprouts.

To help consumers translate the guidelines into practice,
the government released MyPyramid in April 2005.
The pyramid graphic depicts principles of a healthy
diet and lifestyle.

Activity is represented by the steps and the person
climbing them. **Variety** is symbolized by the six color

bands representing grains, vegetables, fruits, milk, meat and beans, and oils. **Moderation** is represented by the narrowing of each food group from bottom to top. The wider base stands for foods with little or no solid fats or added sugars. The narrower top area stands for foods containing more added sugars and solid fats.

Proportionality is shown by the different widths of the food group bands. The widths suggest how much food a person should choose from each group. An interactive tool explaining the pyramid can be accessed through www.mypyramid.gov. Visitors to the site can enter their gender, age and activity level, and receive tailored dietary recommendations based on their specific calorie levels.

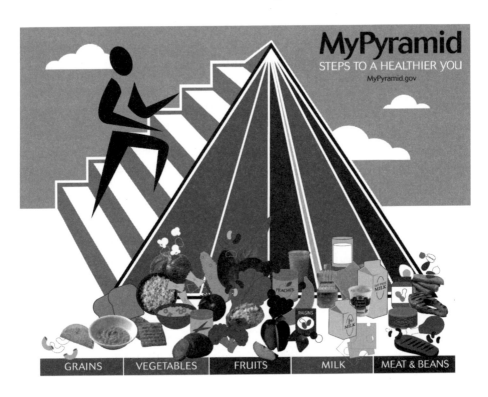

Figuring out how to meet all the nutrition guidelines can seem overwhelming. To help with this process, we've designed menus to illustrate how to follow government recommendations for a healthy diet. Each daily menu below totals 2000 calories, contains 20–35% of calories from fat with less than 10% of calories from saturated fat, and stays within the sodium guideline of 2300 mg daily. The menus also provide the recommended servings of fruits and vegetables. Lycopene is delivered through a variety of fruits and fresh and processed tomato products. Recipes for asterisked items follow the menus.

Sample daily menus

Menu #1
Lycopene: 27.4 mg

Breakfast:

> 2 ounces bran flakes cereal
> 1 fresh-sliced peach
> 1 cup skim milk

Snack:

> 6 ounces unsalted tomato juice
> 1-1/2 ounces walnuts

Lunch:

> Sandwich made with 2 slices whole-wheat bread, 3-ounce grilled chicken breast, lettuce, 2 slices tomato, and 1 tablespoon

low-fat mayonnaise
Fresh baby carrots and red pepper strips
with 1 tablespoon ranch-type dressing
1/2 cup sliced strawberries

Snack:

6 oz. low-fat yogurt
1/2 cup blueberries

Dinner:

Gemelli Pasta with Shrimp and Scallops*
Tossed salad with 2 teaspoons olive oil
and 1 tablespoon Heinz® Red Wine
Vinegar
1/2 cup fresh pineapple
3/4 cup vanilla ice milk

Menu #2
Lycopene: 32.6 mg

Breakfast:

1 medium poached egg
1/2 cup low-fat granola mixed into
6 oz. low-fat yogurt
1/2 cup fresh raspberries

Snack:

Fresh carrot strips

Lunch:

Spinach Salad*
Fire-Roasted Tomato & Garlic Pizza*
Fresh watermelon slice
1 cup skim milk

Snack:

> 4 unsalted Melba toast crackers
> 1 tablespoon chocolate flavored
> hazelnut spread

Dinner:

> Grilled Tuna with Chili Salsa*
> 1 cup steamed green beans
> 1 cup brown rice
> 1 medium pear, sliced
> 1 frozen fruit juice bar

Menu #3
Lycopene: 16.2 mg

Breakfast:

> Omelet made with 1/2 cup egg substitute,
> chopped tomatoes, peppers, onions
> 1 whole-wheat bagel with 1 teaspoon butter
> or soft margarine and 1 teaspoon jelly
> 1/2 cup fresh cantaloupe balls
> 1 cup skim milk

Snack:

> 1/2 cup fresh grapes

Lunch:

> Smashin' Bashin' Bean Soup*
> 1 whole-wheat dinner roll
> 1 medium fresh orange
> 1 cup skim milk

Snack:

> 6 oz. low-fat yogurt
> 1/2 medium banana, sliced

Dinner:

> 3 oz. roasted pork tenderloin
> 1/2 cup fresh zucchini slices cooked with
> 1/2 cup canned crushed tomatoes and
> seasoned with basil
> 1 medium baked potato with 1
> tablespoon light sour cream
> 12 fresh cherries
> 4 chocolate coated graham cracker
> squares

Menu #4
Lycopene: 37.2 mg

Breakfast:

> 1/2 cup oatmeal
> 1/2 cup fresh blueberries
> 1 cup skim milk

Lunch:

> Orzo Salad with Feta and Black Olives*
> 4 oz. sliced chicken breast
> 2 fresh apricots
> 1 cup skim milk

Snack:

> 6 oz. unsalted tomato juice
> 1 oz. almonds

Dinner:

Peppered Vodka Sauce with Penne Pasta*
1/2 cup steamed asparagus
Tossed salad with 2 teaspoons olive oil
and 1 tablespoon Heinz® Red Wine
Vinegar
1 whole-wheat dinner roll
3/4 cup honeydew melon

Menu #5
Lycopene: 11.1 mg

Breakfast:

Strawberry smoothie made with 1 cup
skim milk, 1/2 cup sliced strawberries,
ice cubes, and blended until smooth
1 low-fat oat bran muffin

Snack:

Fresh red and green bell pepper strips

Lunch:

Tomato and Bread Salad with Basil
and Red Onion*
Tuna salad made with 1/2 cup light tuna
canned in water, drained; 1 tablespoon
low-fat mayonnaise, chopped
celery and onions
1 medium apple
1 cup skim milk

Snack:

1 medium fresh orange

Dinner:

> Shrimp Creole*
> 1-1/2 cups cooked brown rice
> 1 cup fresh fruit salad with oranges
> 1 cup skim milk
> 1 frozen dessert pop, double-stick

Menu #6
Lycopene: 19.9 mg

Breakfast:

> 1 cup wheat square cereal
> 2 tablespoons raisins
> 1 cup skim milk

Lunch:

> Pasta E Fagioli*
> 6 wheat crackers
> Sliced tomato with 1 teaspoon olive oil
> and 1 tablespoon Heinz® Red Wine
> Vinegar
> 2 medium plums
> 1 cup skim milk

Dinner:

> 4 oz. grilled salmon
> Honeyed carrots made with 1 cup cooked
> carrot slices, 1 tablespoon honey,
> 1 teaspoon melted butter or soft
> margarine
> Corn on the cob with 1/2 teaspoon liquid
> margarine

2 slices whole-wheat bread

1 cup skim milk

Fresh watermelon slice

Menu #7
Lycopene: 33.6 mg

Breakfast:

6 oz. low-fat yogurt

1 cup cantaloupe balls and strawberry slices

1 slice toasted oatmeal bread with

1 teaspoon jelly

Lunch:

Turkey burger made with 4 oz. grilled ground turkey, served with lettuce, sliced tomatoes, and 1 tablespoon Heinz® Tomato Ketchup on a mixed grain hamburger bun

3 oz. Ore-Ida® French Fries

Fresh tangerine

Snack:

Cucumber salad made with cucumber slices, grated carrots, chopped onions and seasoned with a dressing made with 1 teaspoon sugar, 1 tablespoon Heinz® Apple Cider Vinegar, and 1 teaspoon olive oil.

Dinner:

Chicken & Penne di Genoa*
2 cups fresh baby spinach sautéed
with garlic in 1 tablespoon olive oil
Large fresh pear
1 cup skim milk
1/2 cup raspberry sherbet
2 cream-filled sugar wafer cookies

Recipes

Gemelli Pasta with Shrimp and Scallops

1/4 cup extra-virgin olive oil
1 large Bermuda onion, sliced
4 cloves of garlic, sliced
2 ounces proscuitto, diced
1/2 pound large shrimp, peeled and deveined
1/2 pound sea scallops
1 cup dry white wine
1 cup chicken stock made from Wyler's® Chicken-
flavored Instant Bouillon Granules
1 pinch saffron
2 cups Classico® Cabernet Marinara Sauce
1 pound gemelli pasta, cooked al dente
1 tablespoon hot chili flakes
1 bunch stemmed Italian parsley, chopped

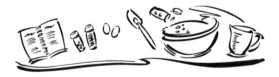

Directions:

In a large heavy pot, heat olive oil over medium high heat. Add onion, garlic and proscuitto, and sauté until softened. Add shrimp, scallops, white wine, chicken stock, saffron, and the Classico® Cabernet Marinara Sauce. Bring to a boil.

Add cooked gemelli pasta to pot and heat through. Add chili flakes and parsley.

Serve immediately.

Serves: 8

Nutrition Information per Serving: 394 calories, 10 g fat, 1.6 g saturated fat, 0 g trans fat, 57 mg cholesterol, 3 g dietary fiber, 727 mg sodium, 10 mg lycopene.

Spinach Salad
Dressing:
    1/3 cup Heinz® Tomato Ketchup
    1/4 cup Heinz® Red Wine Vinegar
    1/4 cup olive oil
    2 tablespoons sugar
    1 tablespoon Heinz® Worcestershire Sauce

Salad:
    1 (10-ounce) bag baby spinach
    1/2 cup fresh mushroom slices
    1 small onion, diced

1 can (15.5 ounces) kidney beans, drained
1 can (8 ounces) water chestnuts, drained and sliced
4 slices cooked bacon, crumbled
1 garlic clove, minced (optional)

Directions:

In a small bowl, mix all ingredients for dressing.
Combine all ingredients for salad in a large bowl.
Just before serving, pour dressing over salad and toss.
Serve immediately.

Serves: 6

*Nutrition Information per Serving: 247 calories, 12 g fat,
2.0 g saturated fat, 0 g trans fat, 6 mg cholesterol,
6 g dietary fiber, 491 mg sodium, 4.1 mg lycopene.*

Fire-Roasted Tomato & Garlic Pizza

2 (12-inch) prepared pizza crusts
1 (26-ounce) jar Classico® Di Siena (Fire-Roasted
Tomato & Garlic) Pasta Sauce
1/2 cup sliced bell peppers
1/2 cup sliced mushrooms
1/2 cup sliced black olives
Chopped fresh basil or oregano leaves
2 cups (8 oz.) shredded fontina cheese

Directions:

Preheat oven to 450°. Place each crust on a pizza pan.
Top with pasta sauce, desired toppings and cheese.

Bake 10 to 12 minutes or until hot and bubbly.
Let stand 5 minutes before serving.

Serves: 16

Nutrition Information per Serving: 117 calories, 6 g fat,
2.7 g saturated fat, 0 g trans fat, 16 mg cholesterol,
1 g dietary fiber, 325 mg sodium, 7.4 mg lycopene.

Grilled Tuna with Chili Salsa
    6-5 oz. fresh tuna fillets
    3 tablespoons olive oil
    1/4 cup lemon juice
    Fresh minced garlic, to taste
    Ground black pepper, to taste

Chili Salsa:
    1 bottle (12 oz.) Heinz® Chili Sauce
    1/2 cup finely chopped green bell pepper
    1/2 cup finely chopped yellow pepper
    1/2 cup finely chopped onion
    2 teaspoons finely chopped cilantro

Directions:

Place the tuna fillets in a shallow pan. Prepare mari-
nade by combining olive oil, lemon juice and enough
minced fresh garlic and pepper to taste. Cover and
refrigerate for at least 30 minutes.

In a medium bowl, combine all salsa ingredients.

When ready to serve, preheat grill to medium-high heat. Grill the tuna on both sides until just cooked through. Do not over cook, or it will dry out.

To Serve:

Place a tuna fillet on a plate and top with the chili salsa. Garnish with fresh cilantro.

Serves: 6

Nutrition Information per Serving: 292 calories, 9 g fat, 1.5 g saturated fat, 0 g trans fat, 67 mg cholesterol, 1 g dietary fiber, 821 mg sodium, 7.4 mg lycopene.

Smashin' Bashin' Bean Soup
    1/4 cup olive oil
    2 large cloves garlic, peeled and chopped
    1 Spanish onion, peeled and chopped
    1 zucchini (about 12 oz.) cut into 1/2-inch dice
    1 yellow bell pepper, stemmed, seeded and cut into 1/2-inch dice
    1 red bell pepper, stemmed, seeded, and cut into 1/2-inch dice
    1 tablespoon chopped fresh basil
    1/2 teaspoon dried thyme
    4 cups vegetable stock made from Wyler's® Vegetable Bouillon
    1 can (16 oz.) plum tomatoes, chopped with their juice
    1/3 cup pitted Calamata olives

2 cans (16 oz. each) Heinz® Vegetarian Beans,
rinsed and drained
4 oz. fresh spinach leaves, trimmed, washed
and coarsely chopped
Freshly ground black pepper, to taste

Directions:

Heat the oil in a large stock pot over
medium heat. Add the garlic and onion,
and sauté until the onion is very tender and
just beginning to brown, about 10 minutes. Add the
zucchini, bell peppers, basil, and thyme. Sauté another
5 minutes. Stir in the vegetable stock, tomatoes with
their juice, and olives. Bring to a boil, reduce the heat,
partially cover, and simmer gently for 25 to 35 minutes. Add the Heinz Vegetarian Beans and spinach,
and cook over medium heat just until the beans have
warmed and the spinach has wilted, about 5 minutes.
Season with freshly ground pepper.

Serves: 12

*Nutrition Information per Serving: 159 calories, 6 g fat,
0.8 g saturated fat, 0 g trans fat, 0 mg cholesterol,
4 g dietary fiber, 664 mg sodium, 3.7 mg lycopene.*

Peppered Vodka Sauce with Penne Pasta

2 tablespoons olive oil
1/2 cup chopped green onions
1/4 pound sliced proscuitto
1 tablespoon minced garlic
1 (26-ounce) jar Classico® Vodka Pasta Sauce
5 plum tomatoes, chopped
Cracked black pepper, to taste
1 (10-ounce) box frozen peas, thawed
Fresh basil, chopped
1 pound penne pasta, cooked al dente
1/2 cup grated Parmesan cheese for topping pasta

Directions:

In a medium saucepan, heat the olive oil and sauté green onions until almost caramelized. Add in proscuitto and garlic. Add in the Classico® Vodka Pasta Sauce and chopped tomatoes. Season to taste with fresh cracked black pepper. Bring to a simmer and cook for 1 minute. Add the peas and the basil, and toss with pasta. Top with grated cheese.

Serves: 6

Nutrition Information per Serving: 585 calories, 20 g fat, 6.2 g saturated fat, 0 g trans fat, 31 mg cholesterol, 8 g dietary fiber, 1162 mg sodium, 19.7 mg lycopene.

Tomato and Bread Salad with Basil and Red Onion

8 ounces stale Italian bread, cut into 2-inch pieces
2 quarts cold water
2 pounds ripe tomatoes, coarsely chopped
(about 5 cups)
1 small red onion, thinly sliced
1 cup loosely packed fresh basil leaves, torn into
bite-size pieces
1/3 cup Heinz® Red Wine Vinegar
1/2 cup extra virgin olive oil
Freshly ground black pepper, to taste

Directions:

Place bread in large bowl. Pour in enough cold water
(about 2 quarts) to cover bread. Soak 5 minutes. Drain
well, squeeze bread to remove as much liquid as possible. Coarsely crumble bread into same bowl. Add
tomatoes, onion and basil. Pour vinegar into small
bowl. Gradually whisk in oil. Season vinaigrette to
taste with freshly ground pepper. Toss salad with
enough vinaigrette to coat.

Can be prepared 8 hours ahead. Cover and chill.
Let stand 1 hour at room temperature before serving.

Serves: 4

*Nutrition Information per Serving: 457 calories, 31 g fat,
4.5 g saturated fat, 0 g trans fat, 0 mg cholesterol,
5 g dietary fiber, 343 mg sodium, 6.8 mg lycopene.*

Shrimp Creole

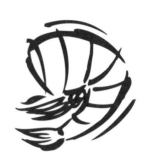

6 tablespoons butter, divided

1 cup julienne onions

1 cup julienne green pepper

2 stalks celery, in julienne strips

2 cloves garlic, chopped

1 bay leaf

2 tablespoons paprika

2 cups diced tomatoes

1/2 cup Heinz® Tomato Ketchup

4 teaspoons Heinz® Worcestershire Sauce

2 tablespoons hot pepper sauce

1-1/2 tablespoons cornstarch

1/2 cup water

3 pounds shrimp, peeled and deveined

Directions:

Melt 2 tablespoons butter in a sauté pan and sauté onion, green pepper, celery, garlic and bay leaf for a few minutes. Add paprika, tomatoes and ketchup. Stir well. Add Worcestershire sauce and hot pepper sauce; simmer until volume is reduced by one-fourth and the vegetables are soft. Mix the cornstarch and water. Stir into the sauce for about 2 minutes to cook the cornstarch.

Sauté the shrimp in the remaining butter until pink and tender, about 5 minutes, stirring constantly. Pour sauce over shrimp and toss to coat well. Serve with fluffy cooked brown rice.

Serves: 8

Nutrition Information per Serving: 250 calories, 10 g fat, 5.8 g saturated fat, 0.3 g trans fat, 275 mg cholesterol, 2 g dietary fiber, 634 mg sodium, 4.2 mg lycopene.

Pasta E Fagioli

2 cups dried cranberry or cannellini beans
5 cups cold water
3 tablespoons olive oil
1/4 pound pancetta, finely chopped
4 large garlic cloves, finely chopped
2 large carrots, peeled and finely chopped
2 large celery ribs, finely chopped
1 large onion, finely chopped
1-1/2 cups canned diced plum tomatoes with juice
8 cups chicken stock made from Wyler's® Chicken-flavored Instant Bouillon Granules Bouillon
Freshly ground black pepper, to taste
1/2 pound small pasta shells, cooked al dente

Directions:

Put the beans in a large saucepan and add the cold water. Bring the water to a boil over high heat; reduce the heat to medium and simmer for about 5 minutes. Turn off the heat and let the beans sit for 1 hour. Drain them and set them aside.

In a 6-quart or larger soup pot, heat the olive oil over medium heat. Add the pancetta and cook, stirring frequently, for 5 minutes. Add the garlic, carrots, celery, and onion and cook, stirring, for 5 minutes longer. Add the beans, tomatoes and chicken stock. Bring to a boil, then reduce the heat and simmer, covered, until the beans are tender, about 1 hour. Season to taste with pepper. Add the cooked pasta shells to the soup and simmer just for a few minutes longer. Ladle the soup into bowls. Top with a liberal grinding of black pepper. Serve immediately.

Serves: 6 as a main course

Nutrition Information per Serving: 573 calories, 16 g fat, 3.8 g saturated fat, 0 g trans fat, 21 mg cholesterol, 13 g dietary fiber, 1249 mg sodium, 5.9 mg lycopene.

Chicken & Penne Di Genoa

    8 ounces penne regate
    1/4 cup flour
    1 teaspoon finely chopped fresh basil
    1 teaspoon finely chopped fresh parsley
    4 skinless and boneless chicken breast halves
    (about 1 pound)
    2 tablespoons olive oil
    1 (26-ounce) jar Classico® Di Genoa
    (Spicy Tomato & Pesto) Pasta Sauce

Directions:

Cook penne regate as package directs; drain. Combine flour, basil and parsley in paper or plastic bag. Add chicken; shake to coat evenly. In a large skillet, over medium-high heat, brown chicken in oil. Remove chicken from skillet; drain. In same skillet, add Classico® Pasta Sauce. Bring to a boil. Return chicken to skillet. Reduce heat. Cover; simmer 15 minutes or until chicken is fully cooked. Serve with hot penne.

Serves: 4

Nutrition Information per Serving: 549 calories, 16 g fat, 2.0 g saturated fat, 0 g trans fat, 63 mg cholesterol, 5 g dietary fiber, 850 mg sodium, 29.5 mg lycopene.

CHAPTER SEVEN

Q & A

Summing Up the Story of Tomatoes, Lycopene and Health

Here are a few frequently asked questions and their answers.

What are free radicals?

Free radicals are highly reactive oxygen byproducts created by normal cell metabolism. Free radicals can also be generated by environmental insults such as air pollution, cigarette smoke and ultraviolet radiation. Free radicals attack cells, causing damage. This damage is thought to be a major cause of many degenerative diseases and the aging process.

What is an antioxidant?

An antioxidant is a substance that has the ability to inactivate harmful free radicals. There is growing scientific evidence that a diet high in antioxidants may protect against certain chronic diseases such as cancer, heart disease and cataracts. Fruits and vegetables are rich sources of antioxidants.

What is lycopene?

Lycopene, one of a family of pigments called carotenoids, gives red tomatoes their color and occurs naturally in fruits and vegetables. Other carotenoids include alpha- and beta-carotene, lutein, etc. Numerous studies suggest that antioxidants such as lycopene may actively inhibit the development of many types of cancer, especially prostate, lung and stomach cancer. Additionally, scientists are studying how consuming tomato products may lower the risk of pancreatic, digestive, breast and cervical cancers. Lycopene and other antioxidants may also play a role in reducing the risk of cardiovascular disease, diabetes and age-related macular degeneration—the most common form of blindness for elderly people in the Western world.

How does it work?

Lycopene is an antioxidant that, once absorbed by the body, helps to protect cells and repair damaged cells. Antioxidants are compounds that fight free radicals in the body and have been shown to inhibit DNA oxidation that can lead to some cancers. Lycopene appears to work together with other compounds in tomatoes to provide beneficial effects.

Does it prevent cancer?

Cancer risk is determined by many factors; diet is an important one. The importance of eating fresh and processed fruits and vegetables as part of a healthy diet has been well recognized for some time. Tomatoes and tomato products are rich in lycopene, a powerful antioxidant that picks up free radicals in the body, and can play a key role in disrupting the process of cancer. And although it is still too early to conclude that any single food can prevent cancer, the research to date is both promising and exciting.

How can I get more lycopene?

The human body does not produce lycopene, but it is readily available through the diet. Minor sources include guava, rosehip, watermelon and pink grapefruit. More than 85% of dietary lycopene comes from tomatoes and tomato products such as juice, soup, sauce, paste and ketchup. Research confirms that lycopene from tomatoes is absorbed much better into the bloodstream if it is first processed vs. fresh off the vine.

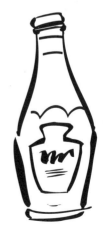

What kind of benefits can I get from consuming sources of lycopene?

As lycopene levels in the blood increase, the levels of oxidized compounds decrease. Growing medical evidence associates high intake of lycopene-rich tomato products with reduced risk of cancers of the prostate, lung and stomach and, possibly, cancers of the pancreas, digestive tract, breast and cervix. Lycopene also may help to prevent macular degenerative disease, the leading cause of blindness in people over the age of 65.

What proof is available that consuming lycopene in tomatoes has these benefits?

Evidence for the role of lycopene in tomatoes in disease prevention comes from tissue culture studies that investigate how cells develop, laboratory studies of animals, population-based studies, and human clinical investigations. Research is strongest for a protective role of tomato products or lycopene for cancers of the prostate gland, lung and stomach. Research is continuing in the areas of pancreatic, colorectal, esophageal, oral, breast and cervical cancers. Scientists have also published studies on the role of tomato product consumption and lycopene in the prevention of cardiovascular disease, diabetes, osteoporosis, and age-related macular degeneration. The web site www.lycopene.org provides ongoing information on results from research studies on lycopene in tomato products.

Can I get the same benefits from eating fresh vs. processed tomatoes?

Red tomatoes are rich in lycopene. However, cooking fresh tomatoes with a little oil will enhance the body's absorption of lycopene. Research confirms that processing tomatoes allows the body to absorb the lycopene more easily. A recent study showed that lycopene is absorbed 2.5 times better from tomato paste than from fresh tomatoes.

How much do I have to eat to make a difference?

To date, no nutritional authority has published recommendations for lycopene intake. More research is needed before lycopene's full public health benefits can be determined and intake guidelines developed. However, based on recent evidence, many health professionals now advocate a diet rich in processed tomato products. Processed tomato products should be part of the nine servings per day of fruits and vegetables suggested by food guidelines promoted in most industrialized countries.

Are there products other than tomatoes that contain lycopene?

Rosehip, pink grapefruit, guava, papaya and watermelon also contain lycopene; however, processed tomato products are usually the highest sources of dietary lycopene.

What research on lycopene is being conducted?

Researchers hope to determine the role tomato products and lycopene play in disease prevention. Current studies are looking at the relationship between dietary lycopene, oxidative stress and cancer risk. The studies will further examine the role of lycopene as an antioxidant in preventing cancer of the breast, prostate, colon, cervix, lung and digestive tract, as well as cardiovascular disease and degenerative diseases of the eye, osteoporosis, diabetes and other diseases.

How can I get the results of future studies?

The web site www.lycopene.org provides ongoing information on lycopene and the research results of studies from around the globe.

Glossary

Antioxidants: Substances that have the ability to inactivate harmful free radicals. There is growing scientific evidence that a diet high in antioxidants may protect against certain chronic diseases such as cancer, coronary heart disease, and cataracts. Substances in food with antioxidant activity that are not vitamins or minerals are sometimes referred to as phytochemicals. Lycopene in tomatoes is an example of a phytochemical with potent antioxidant activity.

Atherosclerosis: A condition in which the lining of the arteries becomes narrow. Caused by an accumulation of fat and other substances, it can lead to coronary heart disease, stroke, and other cardiovascular disorders.

Beta-carotene: The carotenoid in tomatoes with the most Vitamin A activity. It also has antioxidant activity. Once thought to be a major player in cancer prevention, recent scientific studies show less encouraging results, possibly because beta-carotene was studied alone rather than in association with other vitamins and antioxidants.

Botany: The branch of biology concerned with plants.

Calories: Calories are units of energy, commonly used to measure the amount of energy in food and also the amount of energy used by the body.

Carbohydrates: Substances made out of carbon, hydrogen and oxygen, usually sugars and starches. They are a good source of energy. Examples are cereals, breads, pastas, grains, and vegetables such as potatoes.

Carotenoids: The source of Vitamin A activity in tomatoes. Carotenoids are plant pigments, responsible for the bright, rosy color of tomatoes. Carotenoids are fat-soluble, which means they are better absorbed in the presence of oil or fat. There are a number of different carotenoids in tomatoes, such as beta-carotene and lycopene.

Cholesterol: A substance in the blood that helps produce hormones, transport nutrients in the bloodstream, and remove fatty waste products. Where cholesterol is associated with high levels of low-density lipoprotein (LDL), the buildup of fatty plaques on arteries can result. That buildup of plaque may contribute to cardiovascular disease.

Fiber: A mixture of indigestible carbohydrates found in plant foods. It does not supply calories or nutrients, but aids in digestion and elimination. Tomatoes are a source of fiber; people who eat diets high in fiber have a lowered risk of heart disease. Fiber also may protect against some cancers.

Free radicals: Highly reactive oxygen byproducts created by normal cell metabolism. Free radicals lack electrons and try to steal them from other molecules, damaging them. This damage is thought to be a fundamental cause of many degenerative diseases and the aging process. If free radicals attack the molecules involved in normal cellular reproduction, cells may become cancerous. Free radicals can damage the molecules responsible for moving cholesterol through the bloodstream, resulting in the buildup of plaque in the arteries.

Horticulture: The study of growing fruits, vegetables, flowers, and other plants.

Lycopene: The red pigment that gives tomatoes their color, and the predominant carotenoid in tomatoes. Lycopene does not convert to Vitamin A, but may have enormous significance in disease prevention due to its potent antioxidant activity. Lycopene is the most abundant carotenoid in human blood and tissues. Tomatoes are the primary source of lycopene in our diet.

Macular degeneration: A disease in which nerve tissue in the retina deteriorates, leading to gradual loss of sight. It is commonly associated with advancing age.

Oligosaccharides: Non-digestible oligosaccharides are a kind of carbohydrate that is not digested or absorbed by the body. They may help produce healthful bacteria in the digestive tract.

Osteoporosis: A disease in which bones become thinner and weaker; people suffering from osteoporosis are more likely to suffer broken bones.

Oxidation: A chemical reaction involving oxygen. Many scientists believe that, in the body, the oxidation process may create free radicals and damage cells, leading to disease.

Phytochemicals: Hundreds of substances produced naturally by plants to protect themselves from disease. The exact role phytochemicals play in promoting human health is still under investigation, but many phytochemicals have antioxidant activity.

Potassium: Potassium is a mineral that works with sodium to aid the proper functioning of muscles, including the heart.

Proteins: Molecules made up of amino acids. Proteins play many vital roles in the body, including growth and development, cell repair, antibody production, and the production of important chemicals.

Retinol: Retinol is the form of Vitamin A that is derived from animal sources. Carotenoids are the precursors of Vitamin A found in plants.

Vitamins: Essential substances that must be consumed because the body is unable to manufacture them. They are required to maintain health and normal body functions; consuming insufficient amounts may cause disease. Tomatoes are a significant source of Vitamin A and Vitamin C.

Vitamin A: Vitamin A is essential for vision, normal growth, reproduction, and a healthy immune system.
There are two types of Vitamin A — retinoids (preformed Vitamin A found in foods of animal origin) and carotenoids (found in foods of plant origin and converted into Vitamin A). A medium tomato supplies 20 percent of our daily value for Vitamin A.

Vitamin C: Also referred to as ascorbic acid, Vitamin C plays a vital role in combating infection, keeping gums healthy and healing wounds. Vitamin C also is involved in bone health and in regulating blood pressure. One medium tomato meets 40 percent of our daily need for Vitamin C. The vitamin also functions as an antioxidant and may have an additional role in chronic disease prevention, such as cancer and heart disease.

Information in the above glossary includes terms from the Tomato Nutrition Glossary of the Florida Tomato Committee, Copyright 2000, www.floridatomatoes.org/nutrition.html, used with permission from the Florida Tomato Committee.

References

CHAPTER ONE

1. Schröder H, Marrugat J, Vila J, Covas MI, Elosua R. Adherence to the traditional Mediterranean diet is inversely associated with body mass index and obesity in a Spanish population. J Nutr. 2004;134:3355-3361.

2. Vogt TM, Appel LJ, Obarzanek E, Moore TJ, Vollmer WM, Svetkey LP, Sacks FM, Bray GA, Cutler JA, Windhauser MM, Lin P, Karanja NM, for the DASH Collaborative Research Group. Dietary Approaches to Stop Hypertension: Rationale, design, and methods. J Am Diet Assoc. 199;99(suppl):S12-S18.

3. U.S. Department of Health and Human Services and U.S. Department of Agriculture. Dietary Guidelines for Americans, 2005. 6th Edition, Washington, DC: U.S. Government Printing Office, January 2005.

4. Reed J, Frazão E, Itskowitz R. How much do Americans pay for fruits and vegetables? Electronic Report from the Economic Research Service. Available at: www.ers.usda.gov. Accessed June 27, 2005.

5. Lucier G, Lin B, Allshouse J, Kantor LS. Factors affecting tomato consumption in the United States. Vegetables and Specialties/VGS-282/November 2000. Available at: www.ers.usda.gov. Accessed June 27, 2005.

6. Lin, B. Fruit and vegetable consumption. Looking ahead to 2020. Agriculture Information Bulletin 792-7. Available at: www.ers.usda.gov. Accessed June 27, 2005.

CHAPTER TWO

1. Andersen, Craig R. , "Tomatoes," University of Arkansas, Division of Agriculture, Cooperative Extension Service, www.uaex.edu/Other_Areas/publications/HTML/FSA-6017.asp

2. California Tomato Growers Association (CTGA) Web site, www.ctga.org/html/html/FastFacts.html

3. Castleman, Elisabeth Glascon, "Tomato in America," Oct. 28, 2000; AboutFood Web site, www.aboutfood.co.uk/articles/content/ article-222.html

4. Columbia Encyclopedia: Sixth Edition; 2000, www.bartleby.com/65/to/tomato/html

5. Cutler, Karan Davis, "From Wolf Peach to Outer Space: Tomato History & Lore," The Brooklyn Botanic Garden Web site, www.bbg.org/gardening/kitchen/tomatoes/cut-ler.html

6. National Garden Bureau, "Year of the Tomato," www.ngb.org/5/a20.asp

7. Smith, Andrew F., Pure Ketchup; University of South Carolina Press, 1996, p.17-27

8. Winter, Norman, "Tomatoes Rank No. 1 in Mississippi Gardens," Office of Agricultural Communications, Mississippi State University, April 2, 1998 (Available at Web site, www.msucares.com/news/ print/lgnews/msgnews/sg980402.htm)

Chapter Three

1. Andersen, Craig R. , "Tomatoes," University of Arkansas, Division of Agriculture, Cooperative Extension Service, www.uaex.edu/Other_Areas/publications/ HTML/FSA-6017.asp

2. Burpee Seeds & Plants Web site, www.burpee.com

3. California Tomato Growers Association (CTGA) Web site, www.ctga.org/html/html/FastFacts.html

4. Castleman, Elisabeth Glascon, "Tomato in America," Oct. 28, 2000; AboutFood Web site, www.aboutfood.co.uk/articles/content/article-222.html

5. Cutler, Karan Davis, "From Wolf Peach to Outer Space: Tomato History & Lore," The Brooklyn Botanic Garden Web site, www.bbg.org/gardening/kitchen/tomatoes/cutler.html

6. Economic Research Service, U.S. Department of Agriculture, "Vegetables and Melons Situation and Outlook Yearbook," VGS-2005/July 21, 2005.

7. Economic Research Service, USDA. Vegetables and Melons Outlook/VGS-308/April 21, 2005. Available at: www.ers.usda.gov. Accessed June 27, 2005.

8. Encyclopedia Britannica,"Solanaceae," www.britannica.com/bcom/eb/article/0/0,5716,74730+1+72825,00.html?query=tomatoes

9. Lerner, B. Rosie, "1998 Is the Year of the Tomato," Horticulture and Landscape Architecture Department, Purdue University, Web site, www.hort.purdue.edu/ext/98tomato.html

10. Lucier, Gary, "Fresh-Market Tomato Industry Trends," The Tomato Magazine, August 2000, www.freshcut.com/page.cfm?userdate=2000-08-01%2000:00:00&magazine=5

11. National Garden Bureau, "Year of the Tomato," www.ngb.org/scripts/view_article.pl?id=20

12. Nix v. Hedden, 149 U .S. 304 (1893), www.caselaw.lp.findlaw.com/scripts/getcase.pl?court=us&vol=149&invol=304

13. "Tomato: Fruit or Vegetable?," University of Illinois, College of Agricultural, Consumer and Environmental Sciences, Cooperative Extension Service, Horticulture Solutions Series, www.ag.uiuc.edu/~robsond/solutions/horticulture/docs/tomato.html

14. U.S. Department of Agriculture Nutrient Database for Standard Reference, Release 13, November 1999, www.nal.usda.gov/fnic/cgi-bin/list_nut.pl

15. WSU Cooperative Extension, "Tomato Varieties,"
    Gardening in Western Washington, Washington
    State University, www.gardening.wsu.edu/library
    /vege008/vege008.htm

Chapter Four

1. Economic Research Service, USDA. Vegetables and
   Melons Outlook/VGS-308/April 21, 2005. Available at:
   www.ers.usda.gov. Accessed June 27, 2005.

2. Subar, AF, Krebs-Smith SM, Cook A, Kahle LL. Dietary
   sources of nutrients among US adults. J Am Diet Assoc.
   1998;98:537-547.

3. Panel on Dietary Antioxidants and Related Compounds,
   Subcommittees on Upper Reference Levels of Nutrients
   and Interpretation and Uses of Dietary Reference
   Intakes, and the Standing Committee on the Scientific
   Evaluation of Dietary Reference Intakes, Food and
   Nutrition Board, Institute of Medicine. Dietary Reference
   Intakes for Vitamin C, Vitamin E, Selenium, and
   Carotenoids. Washington DC: National Academy of
   Sciences; 2000.

4. U.S. Department of Health and Human Services and
   U.S. Department of Agriculture. Dietary Guidelines for
   Americans, 2005. 6th Edition, Washington, DC: U.S.
   Government Printing Office, January 2005.

5. Laquatra I, Yeung DL, Storey M, Forshee R. Health
   benefits of lycopene in tomatoes-conference summary.
   Nutrition Today 2005;40:20-38.

6. Heber D, Lu Q. Overview of mechanisms of action of
   lycopene. Exp Biol Med. 2002;227:920-923.

7. Porrini M, Riso P, Testolin G. Absorption of lycopene
   from single or daily portions of raw and processed
   tomato. Br J Nutr. 1998;80:353-361.

8. Campbell JK, Canene-Adams K, Lindshield BL, Boileau TWM, Clinton SK, Erdman JW Jr. Tomato phytochemicals and prostate cancer risk. J Nutr. 2004;134:3486S-3492S.

Chapter Five

1. Giovannucci E. Tomatoes, tomato-based products, lycopene, and cancer: Review of the epidemiological literature. J Natl Cancer Inst. 1999;91:317-331.

2. Mills PK, Beeson WL, Phillips RL, Fraser GE. Cohort study of diet, lifestyle, and prostate cancer in Adventist men. Cancer 1989;64:598-604.

3. Giovannucci E, Ascherio A, Rimm EB, Stampfer MJ, Colditz GA, Willett WC. Intake of carotenoids and retinol in relation to risk of prostate cancer. J Natl Cancer Inst 1995;87:1767-1776.

4. Giovannucci E, Rimm EB, Liu Y, Stampfer MJ, Willet WC. A prospective study of tomato products, lycopene, and prostate cancer risk. J Natl Cancer Inst. 2002;94:391-398.

5. Etminan M, Takkouche B, Caamaño-Isorna F. The role of tomato products and lycopene in the prevention of prostate cancer: A meta-analysis of observational studies. Cancer Epidemiol Biomarkers Prev. 2004;13:340-345.

6. Clinton SK. Lycopene: Chemistry, biology, and implications for human health and disease. Nutrition Reviews. 1998;56:35-51.

7. Canene-Adams K, Campbell JK, Zaripheh S, Jeffrey EH, Erdman JW Jr. The tomato as a functional food. J Nutr. 2005;135:1226-1230.

8. Ang E, Miller EC, Clinton SK. Lycopene and carcinogensis. In: Krinsky NI, Mayne ST, Sies H, eds. Carotenoids in Health and Disease. NY: Marcel Dekker, Inc. 2004:409-424.

9. Cook-Mozaffari PH, Azordegan F, Day NE, Ressicaud A, Sabai C, Aramesh B. Oesophageal cancer studies in the Caspian Littoral of Iran: Results of a casse-control study. Br J Cancer 1979;39:293-309.

10. Brown LM, Blot WJ, Schuman SH, Smith VM, Ershow AG, Marks RD, Fraumeni JF Jr. Environmental factors and high risk of esophageal cancer among men in coastal South Carolina. J Natl Cancer Inst. 1988;80:1620-1625.

11. Nkondjock A, Ghardirian P, Johnson KC, Krewski D, and the Canadian Cancer Registries Epidemiology Research Group. Dietary intake of lycopene is associated with reduced pancreatic cancer risk. J Nutr. 2005;135:592-597.

12. Centers for Disease Control and Prevention, National Center for Chronic Diseases Prevention and Health Promotion. 2004/2005 Fact Sheet. The National Breast and Cervical Cancer Early Detection Program: Saving Lives through Screening. Available at: www.cdc.gov/cancer/nbccedp/about2004.htm. Accessed 6-30-05.

13. Public Health Agency of Canada, The Cancer Bureau. Cancer Updates. Breast Cancer in Canada. Available at: www.phac-aspc.gc.ca/publicat/updates/breast-99_e.html. Accessed 6-30-05.

14. Centers for Disease Control and Prevention, National Center for Chronic Diseases Prevention and Health Promotion. Preventing Heart Disease and Stroke. Addressing the Nation's Leading Killers. At a Glance 2005.Available at: nhttp://www.cdc.gov/nccdphp/aag/ aag_cvd.htm. Accessed 6-30-05.

15. Public Health Agency of Canada, Center for Chronic Disease Prevention and Control. Cardiovascular Disease Facts and Figures. Available at: www.phac-aspc.gc.ca/ ccdpc-cpcmc/cvd-mcv/facts_e.html. Accessed 6-30-05.

16. Panel on Dietary Antioxidants and Related Compounds, Subcommittees on Upper Reference Levels of Nutrients and Interpretation and Uses of Dietary Reference Intakes, and the Standing Committee on the Scientific Evaluation of Dietary Reference Intakes, Food and Nutrition Board, Institute of Medicine. Dietary Reference Intakes for Vitamin C, Vitamin E, Selenium, and Carotenoids. Washington DC: National Academy of Sciences; 2000.

17. Arab L, Steck S. Lycopene and cardiovascular disease. Am J Clin Nutr. 2000;7(suppl):1691S-1695S.

18. Kohlmeier L, Kark JD, Gomez-Gracia E, Martin BC, Steck SE, Kardinaal AF, Ringstad J, Thamm M, Masaev V, Riemersma R, Martin-Moreno JM, Huttunen JK, Kok FJ. Lycopene and myocardial infarction risk in the EURAMIC study. Am J Epidemiol. 1997;146:618-626.

19. Fuhrman B, Elis A, Aviram M. Hypocholesterolemic effect of lycopene and beta-carotene is related to suppression of cholesterol synthesis and augmentation of LDL receptor activity in macrophages. Biochem Biophys Res Commun. 1997;233:658-662.

20. Upritchard JE, Sutherland WHF, Mann JI. Effect of supplementation with tomato juice, vitamin E, and vitamin C on LDL oxidation and products of inflammatory activity in type 2 diabetes. Diabetes Care. 2000;23:733-738.

21. Sesso HD, Buring JE, Norkus EP, Gaziano JM. Plasma lycopene, other carotenoids, and and the risk of cardiovascular disease in men. Am J Clin Nutr. 2005;81:990-997.

22. Sesso HD, Simin l, Gaziano JM, Buring JE. Dietary lycopene, tomato-based food products and cardiovascular disdease in women. J Nutr. 2003;133:2336-2341.

23. Mares-Perlman JA, Brady WE, Klein R, Klein BE, Bowen P, Stacewicz-Sapuntzakis M, Palta M. Serum antioxidants and age-related macular degeneration in a population-based case-control study. Arch Ophthalmol. 1995;113:1518-1523.

24. Ford ES, Will JC, Bowman BA, Narayan KM. Diabetes mellitus and serum carotenoids: Findings from the Third National Health and Nutrition Examination Survey. Am J Epidemiol. 1999;149:168-176.

25. Rao LG, Krishnadev N, Banasikowska K, Rao AV. Lycopene I-effect on osteoclasts: Lycopene inhibits basal and parathyroid hormone-stimulated osteoclast formation and mineral resorption mediated by reactive oxygen species in rat bone marrow cultures. J Med Food. 2003;6:69-78.

26. Rao A, Shen H. Effect of low dose lycopene intake on lycopene bioavailability and oxidative stress. Nutrition Research 2002;22:1125-1131.

Index

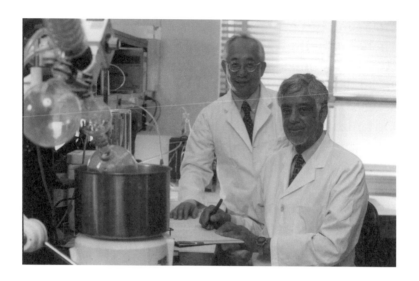

David Yeung, Ph.D.

David Yeung, Ph.D., now a Consulting Nutritionist, retired as Director, Global Nutrition, H.J. Heinz Company April 30, 2005. He received his doctorate degree from the Department of Nutritional Sciences, Faculty of Medicine, University of Toronto.

He was an associate professor in Applied Human Nutrition at the University of Guelph, Ontario, before joining the H.J. Heinz Company. Dr. Yeung remains academically active. He is an Associate Professor in the Department of Nutritional Sciences, University of Toronto, and has been an adjunct and honorary professor in universities in Canada and the People's Republic of China.

Dr. Yeung has published extensively in refereed scientific journals, and he has served on numerous scientific committees in Canada and the U.S.

Dr. Yeung has extensive international experience. He has established nutrition education programs in Australia, Canada, China, the Czech Republic, Hungary, India, Poland, Spain, Thailand, and Russia. He has served as consultant to the Food and Agriculture Organization (FAO), The Micronutrients Initiatives (MI), and the U.S. Agency for International Development (USAID).

In 1997, Dr. Yeung received the Earle Willard McHenry Award from the Canadian Society of Nutritional Sciences for distinguished service in nutrition.

Venket Rao, Ph.D.

Venket Rao, Ph.D., obtained his M.S. and Ph.D. in Food Science from Oregon State University. Dr. Rao is a full professor in the Department of Nutritional Sciences, Faculty of Medicine, University of Toronto. He also is the Director of the Program in Food Safety. He is a member of the Canadian Federation of Biological Sciences, the Society of Toxicology of Canada, and the Bifidous Foundation of Japan.

Dr. Rao's research has established a major focus in the area of diet and cancer with particular emphasis on the role of phytochemicals in human nutrition and health. More recently, he has been investigating the role of oxidative stress and antioxidants in the causation and prevention of chronic diseases. He has studied the role of tomatoes and lycopene in human health extensively and has delivered lectures on this topic nationally and internationally. He has published extensively in scientific journals and participated in many national and international scientific conferences.

Dr. Rao is a member of the Provincial and National Expert Committees in Canada in the areas of food safety and agriculture. He is a member of the National Steering Committee to develop policy guidelines for the Safety of Raw Foods of Animal Origin. He is very active in the Department of Nutritional Sciences as a teacher, research supervisor and as the Undergraduate Coordinator of the Nutritional Sciences Specialist Program. He is frequently sought by the international media for commentary on the subjects of food safety, nutrition and health.

Idamarie Laquatra, Ph.D., R.D.

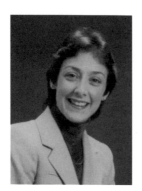 Idamarie Laquatra, Ph.D., R.D., is the Director, Global Nutrition, H.J. Heinz Company. She earned her graduate degrees in nutrition from The Pennsylvania State University. A licensed registered dietitian, Dr. Laquatra has experience in the clinical, academic and business fields. She has extensive training in nutrition counseling, has conducted research in this area, and authored and co-authored articles in peer-reviewed journals and chapters in texts.

Prior to earning her advanced degrees, Dr. Laquatra worked as a clinical dietitian in the hospital and nursing home settings. After completing her Ph.D., she became a postdoctoral fellow in Preventive Cardiology at the University of Medicine and Dentistry of New Jersey. In addition to her postdoctoral studies, she served as adjunct faculty at Montclair State University in Upper Montclair, New Jersey. Her food industry experience began at the H.J. Heinz Company in 1984, where she was employed as Nutritionist for Heinz USA and then Manager of Nutrition for Weight Watchers Food Company. She joined Diet Center, Inc. in 1992 as Vice President of Scientific Affairs and Training. In 1995, Dr. Laquatra began her nutrition consulting business, contracting with clients in both the non profit and for-profit sectors. She rejoined the H.J. Heinz Company as Director, Global Nutrition in 2005.

Dr. Laquatra is also an active member of the American Dietetic Association (ADA). She served as President of the Pittsburgh Dietetic Association, was elected Pennsylvania Delegate, and was appointed Chair of the Advisory Committee of ADA's Food and Nutrition Conference and Exhibition in 2002. The Pennsylvania Dietetic Association presented the Keystone Award to her in 1998 and the Outstanding Dietitian of Pennsylvania award in 2002.